Table of Contents

INTRODUCTION

The Dubrow Diet is a dietary approach developed by Dr. Terry Dubrow and his wife, Heather Dubrow, that focuses on intermittent fasting and cycling between periods of low-carbohydrate and high-carbohydrate eating to promote weight loss and overall health.

A balanced dietary approach that meets individual nutritional needs and health goals is key to supporting overall health and well-being, and the Dubrow Diet may not be appropriate for all individuals, such as those with certain medical conditions or a history of disordered eating.

The Dubrow Diet may be appropriate for individuals who are looking to lose weight and improve their overall health through a structured, cyclical approach to eating. However, it should be approached with caution and under the guidance of a healthcare professional or registered dietitian to ensure adequate nutrition and avoid potential negative effects on health.

Additionally, it is important to note that the Dubrow Diet should not be used as a replacement for medical treatment or medication. A balanced dietary approach that meets individual nutritional needs and health goals is key to supporting overall health and well-being.

CHAPTER ONE

What Is the Dubrow Diet?

The creators of this diet are Dr. Terry Dubrow, a plastic surgeon best known for his role on the show Botched and wife Heather Debrow, a former Real Housewife of Orange County. Their book The Dubrow Diet: Interval Eating to Lose Weight and Feel Ageless is an eating and exercise plan based on the concept of "interval eating." This type of diet focuses on when you eat and promises many health benefits including more normalized insulin and lower blood sugar, fighting off chronic inflammation, activating autophagy (your cells self-cleaning process), reprogramming your cells to use stored fat as fuel, increasing your energy, reaching your goal weight, and rejuvenating your skin and overall appearance.

The basic concept of the book is to focus on "when," "what," and "how much." "When" refers to fasting 12 to 16 hours a day, while "what" and "how much" refer to what to eat outside the fasting window and how much to eat.

One main difference between this intermittent fasting plan and others is the concept of autophagy. The authors tout that when you follow this plan long-term, you will reap the benefits of autophagy, which are similar to the results of plastic surgery. They claim that this is the reason why they both have been able to maintain their appearances. Here's how it works.

What Is the History of a Dubrow Diet?

Heather and Terry Dubrow are the creators of the Dubrow diet. As a husband and wife team who are reality TV stars and wellness experts, the couple wanted to find a more sustainable diet than keto. They first introduced the diet in 2018 with the publication of their book, "The Dubrow Diet: Interval Eating to Lose Weight and Feel Ageless."

The couple developed the Dubrow Diet due to their personal experiences with diet, wellness, and plastic surgery. Heather and Terry noticed that many patients who underwent weight loss surgery struggled with maintaining their weight loss. They saw the need for a more sustainable and health-promoting approach to diet and lifestyle.

The Dubrow Diet quickly gained popularity due to its emphasis on whole, nutrient-dense foods and its use of intermittent fasting to support weight loss. The diet has been widely adopted by people looking to improve their overall health and has received positive reviews from many diet and wellness experts.

How Does the Dubrow Diet Work?

The Dubrow Diet triggers the body's metabolic shift into a state of ketosis, which burns fat for energy instead of glucose. Here's a step-by-step explanation of how the Dubrow Diet works in the body.

Limiting Carbohydrates: Reducing carbohydrates burns fat stores for energy instead of glucose.

Increasing Fat Intake: Healthy fats provide energy and support the body's metabolic shift into ketosis.

Consuming Moderate Protein: High-quality protein supports muscle mass and maintains a healthy metabolism.

Intermittent Fasting: Time-restricted eating reduces insulin levels and improves overall metabolic function.

When the body enters a state of ketosis, the diet targets the liver and other organs, including the brain, muscles, and heart, for increased energy production.

The body's initial reaction to the Dubrow Diet may include increased energy, improved mental clarity, and reduced cravings for sugar and processed foods. It may take two to three weeks to see significant results, such as weight loss and higher energy levels.

The Plan

This plan advocates a low carb diet and includes whole, minimally processed foods including lots of vegetables, healthy fats and lean protein. Fruit, dairy and carbs are allowed, but in very small amounts. Exact recommended foods are listed in the book, along with sample meal plans, recipes and recommended supplements.

The diet is divided into three phases based on fasting window length and allowed foods.

Phase 1

This introductory phase is meant to "reset your internal hunger meter." It is followed for 2 to 5 days and is a 16-

hour fast with an 8-hour window to refuel. Foods that are recommended in this phase include 6 to 12 ounces of lean protein, 1 to 2 servings of healthy fat, 1/2 ounce of nuts or seeds, 1 dairy (or non-dairy) serving, 1 1/2 to 3 cups of non-starchy veggies, 1 small fruit serving, and 1/2 cup of complex carbs. Allowable beverages include water, coffee, tea and "zero calorie" drinks. A savory treat like air-popped popcorn, beef or turkey jerky, or seaweed salad is also allowed.

Phase 2

This weight loss phase is followed until your goal weight is reached. Fasting is 12, 14 or 16 hours a day, depending on how quickly you want to lose weight. Each of the three types of fasting comes with a cheat moment, meal or day. In addition to the foods mentioned in Phase 1, dieters are allowed a bit more complex carbs and healthy fats. Alcohol is also allowed on this phase in moderation (2 drinks per day for men, and 1 drink per day for women).

Phase 3

This is the maintenance phase to be followed long term in order to maintain weight loss and continue to reap the antiaging and disease prevention benefits of autophagy. In this phase, there are 5 days of 12-hours fasts and two 16-hour fasts. You can choose which days to fast for 12 or 16 hours. In addition to the food in Phases 1 and 2, you can opt for one cheat meal a week.

During fasting periods you're allowed beverages and supplements with no sugar and no more than 100 total calories such as coffee, unsweetened tea, water or greens-based supplement drinks. During "refueling" (which is done after fasting) a variety of food is encouraged (which are outlined above), but specific amounts of foods and frequency of consumption are listed in the book. In addition, high intensity interval training is the recommended type of exercise.

What Are The Health Benefits of The Dubrow Diet?

The Dubrow Diet has several potential health benefits, including weight loss, improved insulin sensitivity, increased energy levels, improved digestion, and decreased inflammation.

1. **Weight Loss**: Improve body composition by restricting carbohydrates.
2. **Improved Insulin Sensitivity**: Low-carb, high-fat foods may improve insulin sensitivity and blood sugar control.
3. **Increased Energy Levels**: Fats and protein provide sustained energy.
4. **Improved Digestion**: Emphasizing fiber-rich foods helps improve digestion and support gut health.
5. **Decreased Inflammation**: Nutrient-dense whole foods may help reduce inflammation.

What Are The Health Risks of The Dubrow Diet?

While the Dubrow Diet may offer potential health benefits, it's also essential to consider the potential health risks associated with this diet, including nutrient deficiencies, dehydration, increased cholesterol levels, constipation, and difficulty sticking to the diet.

1. **Nutrient Deficiencies**: Restricting certain food groups may cause nutrient deficiencies, mainly if the diet is not balanced and adequately planned.

2. **Dehydration**: Limiting food intake may lead to dehydration, primarily if adequate water and electrolyte intake are not maintained.

3. **Increased Cholesterol Levels**: High-fat approach may lead to increased cholesterol levels, particularly if you consume unhealthy or processed fat sources.

4. **Constipation**: Restricting carbohydrates may cause constipation, especially if fiber intake is not adequately addressed.

5. **Difficulty Sticking to the Diet**: Strict nature may be challenging for some to maintain, leading to difficulty sticking to the diet and potential weight regain.

How To Do the Dubrow Diet?

Before starting the Dubrow Diet, it's essential to talk with a healthcare professional to ensure that it's safe and appropriate for your health needs and goals.

Here's a step-by-step guide on how to do the Dubrow
Diet:

Familiarize yourself with the phases of the diet: The
Dubrow Diet is in three phases, each with its guidelines
for what to eat and when. Familiarize yourself with the
guidelines for each step, and plan how you will transition
from one phase to the next.

Make a grocery list and meal plan: Make a list of the
foods you will need to follow the Dubrow Diet, and plan
your meals to help you stay on track.

Eat healthy fats and proteins: The Dubrow Diet
emphasizes healthy fats and proteins, such as olive oil,
avocado, nuts, seeds, and grass-fed meats. Incorporate
these foods into your meals, and avoid processed and
unhealthy fats.

Limit carbohydrates: The Dubrow Diet restricts
carbohydrates, particularly refined and processed
carbohydrates. Choose whole food sources of
carbohydrates, such as vegetables and fruit, and limit your
intake of processed and refined carbohydrates.

Incorporate fiber-rich foods: The Dubrow Diet emphasizes fiber-rich foods, such as leafy greens and other vegetables, to support digestion and overall health.

Stay hydrated: The low-carb approach of the Dubrow Diet may lead to dehydration, so it's essential to drink plenty of water and electrolyte-rich beverages.

Monitor your progress: Keep track of your weight loss and how you feel physically and mentally, and adjust your approach as needed to ensure that you achieve your goals.

There isn't a specific limit for the number of calories you should consume on the Dubrow diet. However, if you are focusing on nutrient-dense whole foods that are low in carbs, you will probably be consuming around 1500 calories per day.

The proposed time frame for the Dubrow Diet is not specified, but it's recommended to progress through the phases at a pace that is comfortable and sustainable for you.

The best practices to follow when doing the Dubrow Diet include:

• Planning your meals

• Staying hydrated

• Monitoring your progress

• Adjusting your approach as needed

What Are the Foods That You Can Eat While on A Dubrow Diet?

The Dubrow diet food list includes items you can eat while on the Dubrow Diet vary, depending on the phase of the diet.

1. Proteins: Grass-fed meats, poultry, fish, eggs, and dairy products (in limited amounts)
2. Healthy Fats: Olive oil, avocado, nuts, seeds, and fatty fish
3. Vegetables: Leafy greens, cruciferous vegetables, root vegetables, and other low-carb vegetables
4. Fruits: Berries, apples, and other low-carb fruit
5. Whole Grains: Quinoa, brown rice, and other whole grains (in limited amounts)
6. Legumes: Lentils, chickpeas, and other legumes (in limited quantities)

7. Nuts and Seeds: Almonds, chia seeds, and other nuts and seeds

8. Dairy Products: Greek yogurt, cheese, and other dairy products (in limited amounts)

9. Beverages: Water, herbal tea, and unsweetened coffee and tea

What Are the Foods That You Should Avoid While on a Dubrow Diet?

1. Processed Foods: Chips, crackers, candy, and other processed snacks

2. Refined Sugar: Table sugar, high-fructose corn syrup, and other added sugars

3. Artificial Sweeteners: Aspartame, saccharin, and other artificial sweeteners

4. White Flour: White bread, pasta, and other white flour products

5. Trans Fats: Margarine, shortening, and other products containing partially hydrogenated oils

6. High-Carbohydrate Foods: Pasta, rice, potatoes, and other high-carb foods

7. Alcohol: Beer, wine, and other alcoholic beverages

8. Fried Foods: French fries, fried chicken, and other fried foods

9. Processed Meats: Hot dogs, sausage, and other processed meats high in sodium and preservatives

Who Should Do The Dubrow Diet?

Dubrow Diet is not suitable for everyone. People who are pregnant, breastfeeding, under the age of 18, or have a history of eating disorders should not do this diet.

The diet may benefit people who want to lose weight, improve their overall health, or have digestive issues, such as swallowing disorders or difficulty tolerating normally textured or highly-seasoned foods. People with these issues may find that the low-carb, high-protein approach of the Dubrow Diet helps them feel better and improves their symptoms.

However, it's important to note that the Dubrow Diet should not be the sole treatment for any medical condition and should always be in conjunction with other treatments recommended by a doctor.

Before starting the diet, it's essential to consult a healthcare professional to determine if it's appropriate for you and to develop a safe and effective meal plan.

Recipes for the Dubrow diet are low in carbs and high in protein, and use healthy fats, such as olive oil or avocado, to help keep you on track and achieve your weight loss and health goals. Here are five example recipes for the Dubrow Diet.

1. **Grilled Chicken with Broccoli and Almonds**: This dish features grilled chicken breast served with steamed broccoli and a sprinkle of almond slices for added crunch and healthy fat.

2. **Baked Salmon with Asparagus**: Fresh salmon filets baked in the oven and served with roasted asparagus for a low-carb, high-protein meal.

3. **Turkey and Vegetable Stir-Fry**: Thinly sliced turkey breast is stir-fried with a mix of colorful vegetables and seasoned with a low-carb sauce for a flavorful, satisfying meal.

4. **Egg and Vegetable Breakfast Bowl**: This breakfast bowl features scrambled eggs mixed with diced vegetables, such as bell peppers, onions, and mushrooms, for a high-protein start to the day.

5. **Beef and Vegetable Skewers:** Cubes of lean beef with bell peppers, onions, and mushrooms, and grilled to perfection for a tasty, low-carb meal.

What Is a Sample Dubrow Diet Plan?

Here is a weekly Dubrow Diet plan that anyone can follow.

Day 1

Breakfast: Scrambled eggs with diced vegetables (e.g., bell peppers, onions, and mushrooms) and a side of mixed berries

Lunch: Grilled chicken breast with steamed broccoli and a sprinkle of almond slices

Dinner: Baked salmon with roasted asparagus and a mixed greens salad with olive oil and lemon dressing.

Day 2

Breakfast: Turkey and vegetable stir-fry with a side of mixed berries

Lunch: Grilled shrimp with a mixed greens salad with avocado and lime dressing

Dinner: Beef and vegetable skewers with steamed green beans

Day 3

Breakfast: Egg and vegetable breakfast bowl with a side of mixed berries

Lunch: Grilled chicken salad with mixed greens, cherry tomatoes, cucumber slices, and a low-carb dressing

Dinner: Baked cod with steamed asparagus and a mixed greens salad with olive oil and lemon dressing

Day 4

Breakfast: Greek yogurt with mixed berries and a sprinkle of almonds

Lunch: Turkey and cheese roll-ups with a side of cherry tomatoes and cucumber slices

Dinner: Grilled pork chops with roasted vegetables (e.g., bell peppers, onions, and zucchini)

Day 5

Breakfast: Veggie and cheese omelet with a side of mixed berries

Lunch: Grilled shrimp and vegetable skewers with a mixed greens salad with avocado and lime dressing

Dinner: Baked chicken with roasted vegetables (e.g., bell peppers, onions, and mushrooms)

Day 6

Breakfast: Greek yogurt with mixed berries and a sprinkle of almonds

Lunch: Grilled salmon with steamed green beans and a mixed greens salad with olive oil and lemon dressing

Dinner: Turkey and vegetable stir-fry with a side of mixed berries

Day 7

Breakfast: Veggie and cheese omelet with mixed berries

Lunch: Grilled chicken salad with mixed greens, cherry tomatoes, cucumber slices, and a low-carb dressing

Dinner: Baked beef and vegetable skewers with steamed asparagus

What Are The Facts About Dubrow Diet?
Here are some facts about the Dubrow Diet.

1. **Choose Healthy Options**: This diet encourages the consumption of nutrient-dense, whole foods

2. **Focus on Protein**: Consuming protein-rich foods maintains a healthy metabolism

3. **Eat Slowly and Chew Thoroughly**: You can better tell your body's needs if you slow down and thoroughly process your food, leading to less hunger in the long run

4. **Limit Processed Foods**: Avoid processed foods high in unhealthy fats, added sugars, and artificial ingredients

Heather Dubrow's diet plan emphasizes whole, unprocessed foods and limiting foods high in unhealthy fats. The Dubrow Diet is naturally low in both saturated fat and cholesterol, which can help to reduce the risk of heart disease and other health problems.

How Long Should You Do a Dubrow Diet?

The length of the Dubrow Diet varies based on individual goals and circumstances. You should consult a healthcare professional or dietitian to determine the best plan for you. However, most people make this diet a lifestyle change, continuing the diet for years.

How Long Does It Take for a Dubrow Diet to Show Results?

The length of time it takes to show Dubrow Diet results varies from person to person. However, some people have reported losing weight quickly within the first few weeks of following the Dubrow Diet. You should give it at least two to three weeks to start seeing results.

Does the Dubrow Diet Actually Work?

Limited research on the Dubrow Diet is available, and results may vary for individuals. Some Dubrow diet reviews report success in weight loss and improved overall health. Others may not see significant results.

Is Dubrow Diet Considered a Healthy Diet?

The Dubrow Diet is healthy for those without underlying health problems or eating disorders. Dubrow Diet reviews suggest that this diet is similar to intermittent fasting. It potentially has benefits for reducing inflammation and improving conditions associated with inflammation.

CHAPTER TWO

Fluffy Microwave Scrambled Eggs

Use your microwave to make light and fluffy scrambled eggs for a quick and easy breakfast to start your day. Follow the technique in this recipe for perfect results every time.

Prep Time: 5 mins

Cook Time: 5 mins

Total Time: 10 mins

Servings: 2

Yield: 2 servings

Can You Microwave Eggs?

Of course! We wouldn't be here if you couldn't. This microwave method is hands-off (compared to the traditional stovetop method) and comes together in just a few minutes with three ingredients. What more could you ask for in a shortcut recipe?

How to Cook Eggs In the Microwave

There are plenty of ways to cook eggs in the microwave, but this method for scrambled eggs is perhaps our favorite. You'll find the full recipe below, but here's a brief overview of what you can expect:

Crack the eggs into a microwave-safe bowl or mug, then mix well with milk and salt. Heat the eggs in the microwave for about 30 seconds, remove and beat well, then return to the microwave for another 30 seconds. Repeat until eggs are fully cooked and scrambled.

How Long to Microwave Eggs

Every microwave is different. The process could take anywhere from 1 minute to 2.5 minutes. Just be sure to microwave in 30-second intervals and to beat the eggs between every interval – this way, the eggs will scramble evenly and won't be overcooked.

Microwave Egg Variations

We think this three-ingredient recipe is perfect as it is. But, if you want to dress them up a bit, try one (or more) of these tasty mix-ins:

Cheese

Stir in some shredded Cheddar or Monterey Jack for a cheesy twist.

Ham or Bacon

Diced ham or chopped bacon makes this hearty recipe even more filling.

Veggies

Diced bell peppers, onions, and spinach add color and flavor. To turn up the heat, try jalapeños.

Herbs

Fresh herbs – such as basil, rosemary, oregano, and thyme – lend bright, earthy flavor.

What to Serve with Scrambled Eggs

For a classic breakfast, try pairing these microwave scrambled eggs with Basic Biscuits and Oven-Baked Bacon. You could also make a satisfying Scrambled Egg Sandwich or Breakfast Burrito. With this recipe, it's easy to keep it basic or get as creative as you want. The world is your oyster!

Ingredients

• 4 eggs

• ¼ cup milk

• ⅛ teaspoon salt

Directions

1. Gather all ingredients.

2. Break the eggs into a microwave-proof mixing bowl. Add milk and salt; mix well.

3. Added milk.

4. Pop the bowl into the microwave and cook on high power for 30 seconds. Remove bowl, beat eggs very well,

scraping down the sides of the bowl, and return to the microwave for another 30 seconds.

5. Repeat this pattern, stirring every 30 seconds for up to 2 1/2 minutes. Stop when eggs have the consistency you desire.

6. Serve warm and enjoy!

Nutrition Facts (per serving)

Calories: 141

Fat: 9g

Carbs: 2g

Protein: 12g

Oven Scrambled Eggs

These baked scrambled eggs are light and fluffy and are a snap to put together for a big crowd.

Prep Time: 10 mins

Cook Time: 20 mins

Total Time: 30 mins

Servings: 12

Yield: 1 9x13-inch dish

Ingredients

- ½ cup butter or margarine, melted

- 24 eggs

- 2 ¼ teaspoons salt

- 2 ½ cups milk

Directions

1. Preheat the oven to 350 degrees F (175 degrees C).

2. Pour melted butter into a 9x13-inch glass baking dish.

3. Whisk together eggs and salt in a large bowl until well-blended. Gradually whisk in milk. Pour egg mixture into the buttered dish.

4. Bake uncovered in the preheated oven for 10 to 15 minutes. Stir egg mixture and continue to bake until eggs are set, 10 to 15 minutes more.

Nutrition Facts (per serving)

Calories: 236

Fat: 19g

Carbs: 3g

Protein: 14g

Cauliflower Potato Soup

A yummy cauliflower and potato soup that tastes just like potato soup. Serve topped with shredded cheese.

Prep Time: 20 mins

Cook Time: 3 hrs 15 mins

Total Time: 3 hrs 35 mins

Servings: 4

Ingredients

• 1 head cauliflower, stemmed and chopped

• 2 large red potatoes, cut into 1-inch pieces

• 5 baby carrots, cut into 1/2-inch slices, or more to taste

• 2 teaspoons dried onion flakes, or to taste

• 3 cups water, or as needed

• 1 cube chicken bouillon

• 1 (10.5 ounce) can condensed cream of chicken soup

• ½ cup milk

• ½ (8 ounce) package cream cheese

• 1 tablespoon bacon bits, or more to taste

• ¼ cup chopped fresh parsley, or more to taste

• ½ cup shredded Cheddar cheese

Directions

1. Combine cauliflower, potatoes, carrots, and onion flakes in a pot. Add enough water to cover, then stir in bouillon cube. Bring to a simmer and cook until cauliflower is tender, about 10 minutes.

2. Transfer vegetable mixture and about 1 cup cooking liquid to a slow cooker. Stir in condensed soup, milk,

cream cheese, and bacon bits. Cook on Low for 2 1/2 hours, stirring occasionally.

3. Stir parsley into soup and continue cooking until vegetables are tender and flavors blend, 30 minutes to 1 1/2 hours.

4. Ladle into bowls and top with shredded cheese.

Nutrition Facts (per serving)

Calories: 430

Fat: 21g

Carbs: 48g

Protein: 15g

Creamy Cottage Cheese Scrambled Eggs

Cottage cheese eggs for breakfast are a nice change from regular scrambled eggs. This egg recipe comes out creamy and soft. Perfect with a slice of tomato and turkey bacon for a delicious and fast low-carb breakfast.

Prep Time: 5 mins

Cook Time: 5 mins

Total Time: 10 mins

Servings: 2

Ingredients

• 1 tablespoon butter

• 4 large eggs, beaten

• ¼ cup cottage cheese

• 1 teaspoon chopped fresh chives, or to taste (Optional)

• ground black pepper to taste

Directions

1. Gather all ingredients.

2. Melt butter in a skillet over medium heat. Pour beaten eggs into the skillet; let cook undisturbed until the bottom of the eggs begins to firm, 1 to 2 minutes.

3. Stir cottage cheese and chives into eggs and season with black pepper.

4. Cook and stir until eggs are nearly set, 3 to 4 minutes more.

Nutrition Facts (per serving)

Calories: 224

Fat: 17g

Carbs: 2g

Protein: 16g

Chef John's Summer Scrambled Eggs

Prep Time: 10 mins

Cook Time: 5 mins

Total Time: 15 mins

Servings: 1

Ingredients

1. 3 large eggs

2. 1 pinch red pepper flakes

3. 9 cherry tomatoes, halved

4. 2 tablespoons crumbled feta cheese

5. 1 tablespoon very thinly sliced fresh basil leaves

6. 1 teaspoon olive oil

7. 1 pinch sea salt

Directions

1. Whisk eggs and pepper flakes together in a bowl. Stir in tomatoes, feta, and basil.

2. Heat olive oil in a nonstick skillet over high heat until starting to shimmer. Pour egg mixture into hot oil and cook, without stirring, for 5 seconds.

3. Cook and stir egg mixture until eggs are scrambled and softly set, about 30 seconds. Transfer to a plate and sprinkle with sea salt.

Nutrition Facts (per serving)

Calories: 420

Fat: 33g

Carbs: 10g

Protein: 23g

Basic Fruit Smoothie

This is a great fruit smoothie recipe consisting of fruit, fruit juice, and ice.

Prep Time: 10 mins

Total Time: 10 mins

Servings: 4

Ingredients

- 1 quart strawberries, hulled

- 2 fresh peaches - peeled, pitted, and sliced

- 1 banana, broken into chunks

- 2 cups ice

- 1 cup orange-peach-mango juice

Directions

1. Gather all ingredients.

2. Combine strawberries, peaches, and banana in a blender; blend until smooth.

3. Add ice and pour in juice; blend again to desired consistency.

Nutrition Facts (per serving)

Calories: 118

Fat: 1g

Carbs: 29g

Protein: 2g

Juicy Grilled Chicken Breasts

This grilled chicken breast and marinade is so easy and versatile. My friends and family beg me to make this recipe when the grill is brought out.

Prep Time: 15 mins

Cook Time:15 mins

Additional Time: 30 mins

Total Time: 1 hr

Servings: 4

Ingredients

1. 4 skinless, boneless chicken breast halves

2. ¼ cup lemon juice, plus wedges for serving

3. ¼ cup olive oil

4. 2 teaspoons dried oregano or parsley

5. 1 teaspoon seasoning salt

6. ½ teaspoon ground black pepper

7. ½ teaspoon onion powder

Directions

1. Preheat an outdoor grill for medium-high heat, and lightly oil the grate.

2. Working with one chicken breast at a time, place chicken breast between two sheets of plastic wrap or parchment paper on a cutting board. Using a meat mallet or a rolling pin, gently pound each breast to 1/2-inch thickness.

3. Add lemon juice, olive oil, dried oregano or parsley, seasoning salt, black pepper, and onion powder to a large zip-top bag; add chicken and press out as much air as possible before sealing bag. Gently massage chicken to distribute marinade. Marinate chicken in the refrigerator for at least 30 minutes or up to 12 hours.

4. Preheat grill to medium-high and lightly oil the grate.

5. Place chicken breasts, smooth-side down on preheated grill; cook, covered, until no longer pink and juices run clear, about 5 minutes per side. An instant-read thermometer inserted into the center should read at least 165 degrees F (74 degrees C).

6. Transfer chicken to a cutting board and tent with aluminum foil. Let rest 5 minutes. Serve with lemon wedges.

Cook's Note

I use any leftover grilled chicken (if there is any) for salad the next day.

Nutrition Facts (per serving)

Calories: 139

Fat: 2g

Carbs: 3g

Protein: 27g

Grilled Chicken Marinade

This grilled chicken marinade is the best! It is so flavorful and so simple to prep with easy pantry ingredients. Perfect for any occasion.

Prep Time: 10 mins

Cook Time: 10 mins

Additional Time: 4 hrs

Total Time: 4 hrs 20 mins

Servings: 5

Ingredients

- ¼ cup red wine vinegar

- ¼ cup reduced-sodium soy sauce

- ¼ cup olive oil

- 1 ½ teaspoons dried parsley flakes

- ½ teaspoon dried basil

- ½ teaspoon dried oregano

- ¼ teaspoon garlic powder

- ¼ teaspoon ground black pepper

- 5 skinless, boneless chicken breasts, thinly sliced

Directions

1. Gather all ingredients.

2. Whisk vinegar, soy sauce, olive oil, parsley, basil, oregano, garlic powder, and black pepper together in a bowl.

3. Pour into a resealable plastic bag. Add chicken, coat with the marinade, squeeze out excess air, and seal the bag. Marinate in the refrigerator, at least 4 hours.

4. Preheat grill for medium-low heat and lightly oil the grate. Drain and discard marinade.

5. Grill chicken on the preheated grill until no longer pink in the center, 4 to 5 minutes per side. An instant-read thermometer inserted into the center should read at least 165 degrees F (74 degrees C).

Nutrition Facts (per serving)

Calories: 233

Fat: 14g

Carbs: 2g

Protein: 24g

Cauliflower Pizza Crust

Prep Time: 15 mins

Cook Time: 30 mins

Additional Time: 15 mins

Total Time: 1 hr

Servings: 6

Ingredients

• ½ head cauliflower, coarsely chopped

• ½ cup shredded Italian cheese blend

• ¼ cup chopped fresh parsley

• 1 large egg

• 1 teaspoon chopped garlic

• salt and ground black pepper to taste

Directions

1. Place cauliflower pieces through the feeding tube of the food processor using the grating blade; pulse until all the cauliflower is shredded.

2. Place a steamer insert into a saucepan and fill with water to just below the bottom of the steamer. Bring water to a boil. Add cauliflower, cover, and steam until tender,

about 15 minutes. Transfer cauliflower to a large bowl and refrigerate, stirring occasionally, until cooled, about 15 minutes.

3. Preheat the oven to 450 degrees F (230 degrees C). Line a baking sheet with parchment paper or a silicone mat.

4. Stir Italian cheese blend, parsley, egg, garlic, salt, and pepper into cauliflower until evenly incorporated.

5. Preheat the oven to 450 degrees F (230 degrees C). Line a baking sheet with parchment paper or a silicone mat.

6. Stir Italian cheese blend, parsley, egg, garlic, salt, and pepper into cauliflower until evenly incorporated.

7. Bake in the preheated oven until lightly browned, about 15 minutes.

Nutrition Facts

Calories: 59

Fat: 4g

Carbs: 3g

Protein: 4g

This simple, sensational marinade and sauce for grilled chicken is made with lemon, garlic, rosemary, and butter. Separate the marinade into thirds: 1/3 for marinating, 1/3 for basting, and 1/3 for topping.

Prep Time: 15 mins

Cook Time: 8 mins

Additional Time: 3 hrs

Total Time: 3 hrs 23 mins

Servings: 6

Ingredients

• ½ cup butter

• ½ cup fresh rosemary

• 3 cloves garlic

• 1 lemon, zested

• ¼ cup fresh lemon juice

• 6 (6 ounce) skinless, boneless chicken breast halves

• salt and pepper to taste

Directions

1. In a food processor, blend butter, rosemary, garlic, lemon zest, and lemon juice together. Pour 1/3 of the blended mixture into a small bowl for marinade. Cover remaining mixture, and set aside.

2. Lightly season chicken breasts with salt and pepper. Rub chicken breasts with marinade. Place chicken breasts on a platter, cover, and refrigerate for 3 hours.

3. Preheat an outdoor grill for high heat and lightly oil the grate. Transfer half of the reserved rosemary and lemon mixture into a bowl for basting. Cover remaining mixture, and set aside for topping cooked chicken.

4. Cook chicken breasts on hot grill, basting with rosemary and lemon basting mixture, about 4 minutes per side. An instant-read thermometer inserted into the center should read at least 165 degrees F (74 degrees C). Remove chicken breasts from the grill, and top with remaining rosemary and lemon mixture.

Nutrition Facts (per serving)

Calories: 331

Fat: 18g

Carbs: 2g

Protein: 40g

Grilled Chicken with Rosemary and Bacon

This recipe comes together so easily with minimal prep. Grilled chicken breasts with bacon, garlic powder, and rosemary are cooked to perfection. What could be better? Great with grilled vegetables and rice. Enjoy!

Prep Time: 10 mins

Cook Time: 20 mins

Total Time: 30 mins

Servings: 4

Ingredients

• 4 teaspoons garlic powder

• 4 skinless, boneless chicken breast halves

• salt and pepper to taste

• 4 sprigs fresh rosemary

• 4 thick slices bacon

Directions

1. Preheat an outdoor grill for medium-high heat, and lightly oil the grate.

2. Sprinkle 1 teaspoon garlic powder on each chicken breast and season with salt and pepper. Lay one rosemary sprig on each chicken breast. Wrap bacon around the chicken to hold the rosemary on. Secure bacon with a toothpick or an additional thick rosemary stem.

3. Cook chicken breasts until no longer pink in the center and the juices run clear, about 8 minutes per side. An instant-read thermometer inserted into the center should read at least 165 degrees F (74 degrees C). Stay near the grill to combat any flare-ups from the bacon. Remove the toothpicks before serving.

Nutrition Facts (per serving)

Calories: 208

Fat: 8g

Carbs: 2g

Protein: 30g

Baked Salmon

This baked salmon is a great recipe for beginners. This was my first time making fish and it was a hit. Even my 9-year-old daughter who wouldn't ever dream of eating fish had half of my portion!

Prep Time: 15 mins

Cook Time: 35 mins

Additional Time: 1 hr

Total Time: 1 hr 50 mins

Servings: 2

Ingredients

• 6 tablespoons light olive oil

• 2 cloves garlic, minced

• 1 tablespoon lemon juice

• 1 tablespoon fresh parsley, chopped

• 1 teaspoon dried basil

• 1 teaspoon salt

• 1 teaspoon ground black pepper

• 2 (6 ounce) fillets salmon

Directions

1. Whisk olive oil, garlic, lemon juice, parsley, basil, salt, and pepper together in a medium bowl.

2. Arrange salmon fillets in a small glass or ceramic baking dish; pour marinade over salmon. Cover and marinate in the refrigerator for about 1 hour, turning occasionally.

3. Preheat the oven to 375 degrees F (190 degrees C).

4. Transfer salmon fillets onto a large piece of aluminum foil. Spoon marinade on top and fold up the foil to seal. Place sealed foil packs on a baking sheet.

5. Bake in preheated oven until fish flakes easily with a fork, about 35 to 45 minutes.

6. Serve hot and enjoy!

Nutrition Facts (per serving)

Calories: 613

 Fat: 52g

Carbs: 3g

Protein: 36g

Baked Salmon with Coconut Crust

Many cooks are intimidated by cooking fresh fish and, as a result, miss out on the heart-healthy, brain-boosting, omega-3 fatty acids in salmon. Never fear, though — this recipe for baked salmon with coconut is foolproof!

Prep Time: 10 mins

Cook Time: 15 mins

Total Time: 25 mins

Servings: 4

Ingredients

• 4 (4 ounce) salmon fillets, skin removed

• 1 tablespoon lime or lemon juice

• ½ cup panko (Japanese bread crumbs, available in the Asian food aisle), or substitute dry bread crumbs

• ¼ cup flaked sweetened coconut

• Salt and freshly ground pepper, to taste

• Cooking spray

Directions

1. Preheat the oven to 425 degrees F (220 degrees C).

2. Place salmon fillets on a nonstick baking pan; brush juice on salmon.

3. In a shallow dish, combine panko, coconut, salt, and pepper. Dredge each salmon fillet in panko mixture and

return to the baking pan. Spread leftover crumbs on top of each salmon fillet. Coat with cooking spray.

4. Bake in the preheated oven for 12 to 15 minutes. If desired, put under broiler until crust is golden brown.

Nutrition Facts (per serving)

Calories: 264

Fat: 14g

Carbs: 12g

Protein: 24g

Baked Salmon and Rice

A delicious, healthy dinner of baked salmon and rice with herbs.

Prep Time: 10 mins

Cook Time: 40 mins

Additional Time: 10 mins

Total Time: 1 hr

Servings: 4

Ingredients

• 1 cup brown rice

• 2 ½ cups water

• 1 pound salmon fillet

• ¼ cup orange juice

• 1 teaspoon dried dill weed

• 1 teaspoon dried rosemary

• 1 teaspoon dried basil

• 1 teaspoon dry mustard

• 1 teaspoon lemon pepper

Directions

1. In a saucepan bring 2 1/2 cups water to a boil. Add rice and stir. Reduce the heat, cover, and simmer for 20 minutes.

2. Preheat the oven to 350 degrees F (175 degrees C).

3. In a large pan, add just enough water to cover the bottom of the pan. Place salmon in the pan, pink side up, and arrange cooked rice around the outside of salmon. Drizzle orange juice over salmon and rice.

4. In a small bowl, combine dill weed, rosemary, basil, mustard, and lemon pepper and sprinkle over salmon and rice. Cover with aluminum foil.

5. Bake in the preheated oven for 30 to 40 minutes or until salmon is tender and flaky.

Nutrition Facts (per serving)

Calories: 355

Fat: 14g

Carbs: 30g

Protein: 26g

Spicy Grilled Shrimp

This grilled shrimp recipe is fast and easy to prepare and destined to be the hit of any barbeque. And, weather not permitting, the shrimp cook up great under the broiler, too.

Prep Time: 15 mins

Cook Time: 5 mins

Total Time: 20 mins

Servings: 6

Grilled Shrimp Ingredients

Here are the ingredients you'll need to make this restaurant-worthy grilled shrimp:

• Seasonings: This spicy grilled shrimp recipe is flavored with garlic, coarse salt, paprika, and cayenne pepper.

• Oil: Olive oil locks in the moisture and gives the seasonings something to stick to.

• Lemon: You'll need lemon juice for flavor and lemon wedges for the garnish.

• Shrimp: Buy your shrimp pre-peeled and deveined or do it yourself at home.

How to Cook Shrimp On the Grill

Here's a brief overview of what you can expect when you make spicy grilled shrimp recipe:

1. Make a paste with the garlic, oil, seasonings, and lemon juice.

2. Toss the shrimp in the garlic paste until evenly coated.

3. Grill the shrimp, then garnish with lemon wedges before serving.

How Long to Grill Shrimp

On a lightly oiled grill grate over medium heat, the shrimp should be fully cooked after about 2-3 minutes on each side. You'll know the shrimp is done when it's opaque.

How to Store Grilled Shrimp Leftovers

Store your grilled shrimp leftovers in an airtight container in the refrigerator for up to three days. Put them to good use by tossing them in one of our favorite Shrimp Salads.

Ingredients

• 1 large clove garlic

- 1 teaspoon coarse salt

- 1 teaspoon paprika

- ½ teaspoon cayenne pepper

- 2 tablespoons olive oil

- 2 teaspoons lemon juice

- 2 pounds large shrimp, peeled and deveined

- 8 wedges lemon, for garnish

Directions

1. Gather the ingredients. Preheat a grill for medium heat.

2. Crush garlic and salt together in a small bowl with a fork.

3. Mix in paprika and cayenne. Stir in olive oil and lemon juice to form a paste.

4. Combine garlic paste and shrimp in a large bowl and toss until shrimp are evenly coated.

5. Lightly oil the grill grate. Grill shrimp until opaque, 2 to 3 minutes per side.

6. Transfer to a serving dish, garnish with lemon wedges, and serve.

Nutrition Facts (per serving)

Calories: 164

Fat: 6g

Carbs: 3g

Protein: 25g

Honey Grilled Shrimp

Easy and delicious honey grilled shrimp! Onions, peppers, and mushrooms are perfect when alternated with shrimp on the skewers. Just cut into bite-sized pieces and add them to the marinade with the shrimp. Serve with rice and a salad.

Prep Time: 15 mins

Cook Time: 5 mins

Additional Time: 1 hr

Total Time: 1 hr 20 mins

Servings: 3

Ingredients

• ½ teaspoon garlic powder

• ¼ tablespoon ground black pepper

• ⅓ cup Worcestershire sauce

• 2 tablespoons dry white wine

• 2 tablespoons Italian-style salad dressing

• 1 pound large shrimp, peeled and deveined with tails attached

• ¼ cup honey

• ¼ cup butter, melted

• 2 tablespoons Worcestershire sauce

• skewers

Directions

• In a large bowl, mix together garlic powder, black pepper, 1/3 cup Worcestershire, wine, and dressing; add shrimp and toss to coat. Cover and marinate in the refrigerator for 1 hour.

• Preheat the grill to high heat. Thread shrimp onto skewers, piercing once near the tail and once near the head. Discard marinade.

• In a small bowl, stir together honey, melted butter, and remaining 2 tablespoons Worcestershire sauce. Set aside for basting.

• Lightly oil the grill grate. Grill shrimp for 2 to 3 minutes per side, or until opaque. Baste occasionally with the honey-butter sauce while grilling.

Nutrition Facts (per serving)

Calories: 434

Fat: 20g

Carbs: 33g

Protein: 30g

Delicious spicy marinated shrimp. Easy on indoor or outdoor grill. I serve this with yellow rice and/or baked potatoes. I also put an extra shot of hot pepper sauce on the rice, love it spicy!

Prep Time: 15 mins

Cook Time: 5 mins

Additional Time: 30 mins

Total Time: 50 mins

Servings: 6

Yield: 6 servings

Ingredients

• 3 cloves garlic, minced

• 2 chipotle peppers in adobo sauce, chopped

• 1 lemon, juiced

• 1 tablespoon olive oil

• 1 tablespoon paprika

- 1 teaspoon chopped fresh cilantro (Optional)

- 1 teaspoon kosher salt

- ½ teaspoon cracked black pepper

- ½ teaspoon crushed red pepper flakes

- ¼ teaspoon cayenne pepper

- 2 pounds uncooked medium shrimp, peeled and deveined

- wooden or metal skewers

Directions

1. Mix together the garlic, chipotle peppers, lemon juice, olive oil, paprika, cilantro, kosher salt, black pepper, red pepper flakes, and cayenne pepper in a bowl. Stir in the shrimp, and mix well to thoroughly coat. Marinate for 30 minutes in refrigerator.

2. Preheat an outdoor grill for medium-high heat, and lightly oil the grate.

3. Remove the shrimp from the marinade, and discard excess marinade. Thread about 5 shrimp per skewer, and

grill on the preheated grill until the shrimp turn pink and opaque in the center, about 2 minutes per side.

Nutrition Facts (per serving)

Calories: 150

Fat: 4g

Carbs: 4g

Protein: 25g

Grilled Garlic and Herb Shrimp

This is an easy recipe to prep for grilled shrimp using a marinade made with fresh garlic, lemon juice, olive oil, Italian herb seasoning, brown sugar, and paprika. Every time I make it I have people begging me for the recipe.

Prep Time: 10 mins

Cook Time: 5 mins

Additional Time: 2 hrs

Total Time: 2 hrs 15 mins

Servings: 4

Ingredients

• 2 teaspoons ground paprika

• 2 tablespoons fresh minced garlic

• 2 teaspoons Italian seasoning, or to taste

• 2 tablespoons fresh lemon juice

• ¼ cup olive oil

• ½ teaspoon ground black pepper

• 2 teaspoons dried basil leaves

• 2 tablespoons brown sugar, packed

• 2 pounds large shrimp (21-25 per pound), peeled and deveined

Directions

1. Whisk the paprika, garlic, Italian seasoning, lemon juice, olive oil, pepper, basil, and brown sugar together in a bowl until thoroughly blended.

2. Stir in the shrimp, and toss to evenly coat with the marinade. Cover and refrigerate at least 2 hours, turning once.

3. Preheat an outdoor grill for medium-high heat. Lightly oil grill grate, and place about 4 inches from heat source.

4. Remove shrimp from marinade, drain excess, and discard marinade.

5. Place shrimp on preheated grill and cook, turning once, until opaque in the center, 5 to 6 minutes. Serve immediately.

Nutrition Facts (per serving)

Calories: 336

Fat: 16g

Carbs: 10g

Protein: 38g

This grilled chicken salad is both beautiful in presentation and taste. You can use fresh berries in summer (strawberries, blueberries, raspberries, or blackberries) and orange segments in winter. This terrific salad recipe will bring rave reviews any time of the year!

Prep Time: 15 mins

Cook Time: 20 mins

Total Time: 35 mins

Servings: 6

Ingredients

• 1-pound skinless, boneless chicken breast halves

• ½ cup pecans

• ⅓ cup red wine vinegar

• ½ cup white sugar

• 1 cup vegetable oil

• ½ onion, minced

- 1 teaspoon ground mustard

- 1 teaspoon salt

- ¼ teaspoon ground white pepper

- 2 heads Bibb lettuce - rinsed, dried and torn

- 1 cup sliced fresh strawberries

Directions

1. Preheat the grill to high heat. Lightly oil the grill grate.

2. Grill chicken until juices run clear, about 8 minutes per side. Remove from heat, cool, and slice. Set aside.

3. Meanwhile, place pecans in a dry skillet over medium-high heat. Cook pecans, stirring frequently, until fragrant, about 8 minutes. Remove from heat and set aside.

4. To make the dressing: Combine red wine vinegar, sugar, vegetable oil, onion, mustard, salt, and pepper in a blender. Process until smooth.

5. Arrange lettuce on serving plates. Top with grilled chicken slices, strawberries, and pecans. Drizzle with dressing to serve.

Nutrition Facts (per serving)

Calories: 567

Fat: 46g

Carbs: 23g

Protein: 18g

Grilled Chicken Salad Sandwich

This is a great way to use leftover grilled chicken breasts from dinner the night before. I like it on wheat. My husband likes it on sourdough.

Prep Time: 15 mins

Total Time: 15 mins

Servings: 4

Yield: 4 sandwiches

Ingredients

• 1 cup mayonnaise

• ⅛ teaspoon ground black pepper

- ⅛ teaspoon garlic powder

- ⅛ teaspoon celery salt

- 4 cups chopped leftover grilled chicken

- 2 celery stalks, sliced

- ½ cup sweetened dried cranberries

- ⅔ cup salted cashews

- 8 slices bread, toasted

- 4 tablespoons mayonnaise

- 4 large red leaf lettuce leaves

- 1 ripe tomato, sliced

Directions

1. Whisk together 1 cup of mayonnaise, pepper, garlic powder, and celery salt until combined. Combine the chicken, celery, cranberries, and cashews in a large bowl. Pour the mayonnaise mixture over the chicken mixture and stir until evenly combined.

2. Spread 1/2 tablespoon of mayonnaise on each slice of toasted bread. Divide the chicken salad between four of the slices of toast; top each with a lettuce leaf and a slice of tomato. Complete each sandwich with the remaining toast slices.

Nutrition Facts (per serving)

Calories: 1078

Fat: 77g

Carbs: 50g

Protein: 47g

Amy's Barbecue Chicken Salad

This recipe for barbecue chicken salad is very similar to one at a popular restaurant near my house. I loved it there and decided to make it at home. Now it's one of my favorite salads to make!

Prep Time: 20 mins

Cook Time: 15 mins

Additional Time: 10 mins

Total Time: 45 mins

Servings: 8

Ingredients

• 2 skinless, boneless chicken breast halves

• 1 head red leaf lettuce, rinsed and torn

• 1 head green leaf lettuce, rinsed and torn

• 1 fresh tomato, chopped

• 1 bunch cilantro, chopped

• 1 (15.25 ounce) can whole kernel corn, drained

• 1 (15 ounce) can black beans, drained

• 1 (2.8 ounce) can French fried onions

• ½ cup ranch dressing

• ½ cup barbecue sauce

Directions

1. Preheat the grill for high heat and lightly oil the grate.

2. Cook chicken on the preheated grill until the juices run clear, about 6 minutes per side. An instant-read thermometer inserted into the center should read at least 165 degrees F (74 degrees C). Remove from heat, cool, and slice.

3. In a large bowl, mix lettuces, tomato, cilantro, corn, and black beans. Top with grilled chicken slices and French fried onions.

4. In a small bowl, mix ranch dressing and barbecue sauce together. Serve on the side as a dipping sauce or toss with the salad to coat.

Nutrition Facts (per serving)

Calories: 301

Fat: 14g

Carbs: 32g

Protein: 12g

These grilled pork chops are simple to prepare with an easy marinade you can make in the morning for a tasty dinner that cooks on the grill in just 10 minutes.

Prep Time: 5 mins

Cook Time: 10 mins

Additional Time: 2 hrs

Total Time: 2 hrs 15 mins

Servings: 6

Ingredients

- ½ cup water

- ⅓ cup light soy sauce

- ¼ cup vegetable oil

- 3 tablespoons lemon pepper seasoning

- 2 teaspoons minced garlic

- 6 boneless pork loin chops, trimmed of fat

Directions

1. Mix water, soy sauce, vegetable oil, lemon-pepper seasoning, and garlic in a deep bowl; add pork chops and toss to coat. Marinate in the refrigerator for at least 2 hours.

2. Preheat an outdoor grill for medium-high heat and lightly oil the grate.

3. Remove pork chops from the marinade and shake off excess; discard the remaining marinade.

4. Cook the pork chops on the preheated grill until no longer pink in the center, 5 to 6 minutes per side. An instant-read thermometer inserted into the center should read 145 degrees F (63 degrees C).

5. Serve hot and enjoy!

Nutrition:

The nutrition data for this recipe includes the full amount of the marinade ingredients. The actual amount of the marinade consumed will vary.

Nutrition Facts (per serving)

Calories: 380

Fat: 22g

Carbs: 2g

Protein: 41g

World's Best Honey Garlic Pork Chops
A quick and simple grilled pork chop that everyone will love featuring a simple and easy glaze made with ketchup, honey, soy sauce, and garlic.

Prep Time: 10 mins

Cook Time: 20 mins

Total Time: 30 mins

Servings: 6

Ingredients

• ½ cup ketchup

• 2 ⅔ tablespoons honey

- 2 tablespoons low-sodium soy sauce

- 2 cloves garlic, crushed

- 6 (4 ounce) (1-inch thick) pork chops

Directions

1. Preheat grill for medium heat and lightly oil the grate. Gather ingredients.

2. Four raw, bone-in pork chops on a baking sheet with 4 small bowls of ingredients on the side

3. Whisk ketchup, honey, soy sauce, and garlic together in a bowl to make a glaze.

4. Overhead view of brown sauce inside of a clear glass bowl and a hand with a whisk stirring said sauce

5. Sear the pork chops on both sides on the preheated grill. Lightly brush glaze onto each side of the chops as they cook; grill until no longer pink in the center, about 7 to 9 minutes per side. An instant-read thermometer inserted into the center should read 145 degrees F (63 degrees C).

6. Overhead view of 4 pork chops on a griddle. Brush with sauce on the surface of one of the pork chops.

7. Serve hot and enjoy!

Nutrition Facts (per serving)

Calories: 290

Fat: 13g

Carbs: 14g

Protein: 30g

Celery Soup
Recipe Summary

Prep:30 mins

Cook:1 hr

Additional:20 mins

Total:1 hr 50 mins

Servings:6

Yield:6 servings

Ingredients

• 3 tablespoons olive oil, divided, or to taste

• 1 large onion, chopped

• 2 carrots, peeled and chopped, or more to taste

• 1 leek, thinly sliced

• 4 cloves garlic, peeled and chopped

• 6 cups diced celery

• 1 quart chicken bone broth

• 1 ½ pounds baby yellow potatoes, peeled

• 1 small bunch fresh parsley

• 1 teaspoon dried thyme, or to taste

• ½ teaspoon salt-free seasoning blend

• salt and ground black pepper to taste

Directions

Step 1

Heat 2 tablespoons olive oil in a frying pan over medium heat. Add onion, carrots, and leek; cook until soft, about 5 minutes. Add garlic; cook for 1 minute. Transfer to a soup pot.

Step 2

Heat remaining olive oil in the same frying. Saute celery to release some of the moisture, about 10 minutes.

Step 3

Transfer celery to the soup pot. Add chicken broth and potatoes. Cut parsley into the pot using kitchen scissors. Season soup with thyme, seasoning blend, salt, and pepper. Increase heat to medium-high and bring to a rolling simmer.

Step 4

Reduce heat and simmer until carrots, celery, and potatoes are soft enough to easily puree, about 30 minutes. Avoid cooking vegetables until mushy. Remove from heat and cool for about 20 minutes.

Step 5

Puree soup with an immersion blender. Simmer over low heat until heated through, 10 to 15 minutes. Serve immediately or let flavors meld overnight and serve the next day.

Cook's Notes:

Feel free to add whatever seasonings you like.

To puree soup in a food processor or blender, divide it into 2 batches.

Nutrition Facts

Per Serving: 208 calories; protein 4.6g; carbohydrates 32.1g; fat 7.7g; cholesterol 0.5mg; sodium 607.9mg.

Pepper And Onion Medley
Recipe Summary

Serves: 3 Time to make: 30 minute

Ingredients

- 1 orange bell pepper

- 1 yellow bell pepper
- 2 red bell peppers
- 1/2 of a medium sized onion
- 6 basil leaves Sea salt
- Black pepper
- Extra virgin olive oil

Directions

Slice your bell peppers and onion into thin pieces. Heat a large pan to medium heat (No. 5), and once the pan is hot, add some olive oil to the pan. Then add your peppers, onions, and season everything with some salt and black pepper. Stir everything continuously for 5 minutes, then put the lid on the pan, and reduce the heat to medium-low (No. 2) for 15-20 minutes. The peppers and onions are done when a chef's knife penetrates a pepper by its own weight. Remove the pan from the stove, chop up the basil and add it to the dish. Correct seasoning with salt and pepper if need be.

Serves: 1 Time to make: <10 minutes

Ingredients

• 3-4 large kale stalks

• 1 avocado

• 1 clove of garlic

• 4-5 fresh basil leaves

• Sea salt

• Black pepper

• Extra virgin olive oil

Directions

Remove the stem from your kale stalks and chops the kale into bite sized pieces. Steam the kale for 2 minutes. Grab a mixing bowl and add the meat of the avocado to the bowl. Use a potato masher to completely mash the avocado. Chop your basil leaves and add them to the bowl. Use a garlic press and add your garlic to the bowl. Once your kale is done, add it to the bowl along with salt, black pepper, and a quick splash of olive oil. Use a spoon to mix everything together. Correct seasoning if need be.

Serves: 2 Time to make: 30 minutes

Ingredients

• 4 free-range eggs

• 1 medium yellow onion

• 2 pints of cherry tomatoes

• 1 handful of fresh basil

• Sea salt

• Black pepper

• Extra virgin olive oil

Directions

First start by slicing the onion into thin slices and the cherry tomatoes into halves -- chop the basil, but not too much. Heat a pan to medium heat (No. 5) on the stove.

Once the pan is hot, add olive oil to the pan and gently place the onion into the pan away from your position. Add a little sat and pepper. Cook the onions for about 5 minutes or unit they're just about transparent and then add the tomatoes and fresh basil. Add a little more salt and pepper. Stir everything together and continue to do so for about 5 minutes or until the tomatoes begin to wilt -- don't overcook the onions! Once the tomatoes begin to wilt, crack the eggs on top of everything -- don't stir -- place a lid on the pan, reduce the heat to low (No. 1), and let the dish sit for about 4-5 minutes to cook the eggs. If you like runny eggs, leave the lid on for 1-3 minutes instead. Remove from the stove and let it sit to cool for 5 minutes. Correct seasoning if need be.

Avocado Egg Salad

Recipe Summary

Serves: 2 Time to make: 20 minutes

Ingredients

• 4 hard boiled eggs

• 1 avocado

• 2 tsp of apple cider vinegar

• 1/8 tsp of powdered mustard

• Sea salt

• Black pepper

Directions

Bring a small pot to a roaring boil and place eggs in [after the water boils] for 9 to 10 minutes. Once your eggs are done, run them under cold water and let them sit for 5 minutes. Grab a bowl, add the whole avocado and mash it up with a fork or potato masher. Now peel your eggs and either run them through an egg slicer twice -- once vertically and horizontally -- or use a knife to dice them up. Add the eggs to the bowl along with the mustard, apple cider vinegar, and salt and pepper to taste.

Recipe summary

Prep: 10 mins

Total: 10 mins

Servings: 1

Yield: 1 smoothie

Ingredients

- ½ cup 2% milk

- ½ cup orange juice

- ½ mango - peeled, seeded, and cut into chunks

- ½ fresh peach - peeled, pitted, and sliced

- ¼ cup fresh pineapple chunks

- 2 strawberries

Directions

Step 1

Blend milk, orange juice, mango, peach, pineapple, and strawberries together in a blender until smooth.

Cook's Note:

If this not smooth enough, add milk and orange juice until desired consistency is reached.

Nutrition Facts

Per Serving: 225 calories; protein 5.8g; carbohydrates 46.4g; fat 3.1g; cholesterol 9.8mg; sodium 55.9mg.

Mango Cherry Smoothie
Prep: 10 mins

Total: 10 mins

Servings: 2

Yield: 2 servings

Ingredients

• 2 cups pitted cherries

• 1 cup chopped mango

- 1 cup water

- 1 cup ice cubes

Directions

Step 1

Blend cherries, mango, water, and ice cubes together in a blender until smooth.

Cook's Note:

For a thicker smoothie, add less water.

Nutrition Facts

Per Serving: 158 calories; protein 2.2g; carbohydrates 38g; fat 1.6g; sodium 8.9mg.

Tangy Broccoli
Prep: 10 mins

Cook: 10 mins

Total: 20 mins

Servings: 4

Yield: 4 servings

Ingredients

• 1 large head broccoli, cut into florets

• 2 tablespoons prepared Dijon-style mustard

• 4 ounces process cheese food

Directions

Step 1

Steam broccoli until tender-crisp.

Step 2

Toss broccoli with mustard, then melt the cheese over the broccoli in a microwave for 1 minute on HIGH. Stir and serve.

Nutrition Facts

Per Serving: 143 calories; protein 8.6g; carbohydrates 7.6g; fat 9.2g; cholesterol 26.6mg; sodium 637.4mg.

Prep: 10 mins

Additional: 3 hrs

Total: 3 hrs 10 mins

Servings: 6

Yield: 6 servings

Ingredients

• ½ cup olive oil

• ¼ cup red wine vinegar

• 1 (.7 ounce) package dry Italian salad dressing mix (such as Good Seasons®)

• 3 heads broccoli, cut into florets

Directions

Step 1

Combine olive oil, red wine vinegar, and Italian dressing mix in a sealable container; shake vigorously.

Step 2

Place broccoli in a plastic storage container, cover with marinade, and refrigerate, stirring occasionally, for at least 3 hours.

Nutrition Facts

Per Serving: 221 calories; protein 4.2g; carbohydrates 12.3g; fat 18.6g; sodium 580mg.

Steamed Broccoli
Prep: 10 mins

Cook: 5 mins

Total: 15 mins

Servings: 2

Yield: 2 servings

Ingredients

• 1 head broccoli, cut into florets

• 1 slice cooked bacon, chopped

• 1 tablespoon butter

• salt and ground black pepper to taste

Directions

Step 1

Place a steamer insert into a saucepan and fill with water to just below the bottom of the steamer. Bring water to a boil. Add broccoli, cover, and steam until tender, 3 to 5 minutes.

Step 2

Mix steamed broccoli, bacon, butter, salt, and pepper together in a bowl.

Nutrition Facts

Per Serving: 102 calories; protein 4.3g; carbohydrates 10g; fat 6.3g; cholesterol 15.3mg; sodium 90.4mg.

CONCLUSION

The Dubrow Diet is a structured, cyclical dietary approach that emphasizes intermittent fasting and cycling between periods of low-carbohydrate and high-carbohydrate eating to promote weight loss and overall health. While it may offer potential benefits, it should be approached with caution and under the guidance of a healthcare professional or registered dietitian to ensure adequate nutrition and avoid potential negative effects on health.

The Dubrow Diet itself doesn't have scientific merit behind it. However, intermittent fasting does have some substantiating research primarily in animal studies. To date, there is much debate around the concept of intermittent fasting and weight loss and there is uncertainty as to whether it's the fasting or the calorie restriction that leads to weight loss. The diet encourages a variety of foods including lots of vegetables, but not all foods are encouraged in the amounts needed daily by the body leaving room for potential nutrient deficiencies.

When it comes to diets, there is no "one size fits all," but you certainly do need to take in all the nutrients that your body needs.